This Book Belongs To

NAME	
ADDRESS	
CITY	
STATE	
E-MAIL	
PHONE	
CELL	

My Cat

NAME	
BREED	
BIRTH DATE	
COLOR	
VET'S NAME	
VET'S PHONE	

D1530663

Cat Picture

About My Cat

	Information	Add'l Details
Spayed / Neutered	Yes / No	
Allergies	Yes / No	
Illnesses	Yes / No	
Injuries	Yes / No	
Micrichip	Yes / No	
Cat Tag Registration	Yes / No	
Breed Registration	Yes / No	
Identifying Marks	Yes / No	
Anxiety Triggers	Yes / No	
Attack Triggers	Yes / No	
Behaviour Issues	Yes / No	
Favorite Games/Toys	Yes / No	
Blood Type		
Food Type		
Food Name		
Feeding Time		
Medications		
Notes		

Vet Visits

Date	
Vet Name	
E-Mail	
Phone	
Reason For Visit	
Tests Done	
Diagnosis	
Treatment	
Mediction	
SHOT / VACCINATIONS	
WEIGHT	

Vet Visits

Date	
Vet Name	
E-Mail	
Phone	
Reason For Visit	
Tests Done	
Diagnosis	
Treatment	
Mediction	
SHOT / VACCINATIONS	
WEIGHT	

Vet Visits

Date	
Vet Name	
E-Mail	
Phone	
Reason For Visit	
Tests Done	
Diagnosis	
Treatment	
Mediction	
SHOT / VACCINATIONS	
WEIGHT	

Vet Visits

Date	
Vet Name	
E-Mail	
Phone	
Reason For Visit	
Tests Done	
Diagnosis	
Treatment	
Mediction	
SHOT / VACCINATIONS	
WEIGHT	

Vet Visits

Date	
Vet Name	
E-Mail	
Phone	
Reason For Visit	
Tests Done	
Diagnosis	
Treatment	
Mediction	
SHOT / VACCINATIONS	
WEIGHT	

Vet Visits

Date	
Vet Name	
E-Mail	
Phone	
Reason For Visit	
Tests Done	
Diagnosis	
Treatment	
Mediction	
SHOT / VACCINATIONS	
WEIGHT	

Vet Visits

Date	
Vet Name	
E-Mail	
Phone	
Reason For Visit	
Tests Done	
Diagnosis	
Treatment	
Mediction	
SHOT / VACCINATIONS	
WEIGHT	

Vet Visits

Date	
Vet Name	
E-Mail	
Phone	
Reason For Visit	
Tests Done	
Diagnosis	
Treatment	
Mediction	
SHOT / VACCINATIONS	
WEIGHT	

Vet Visits

Date	
Vet Name	
E-Mail	
Phone	
Reason For Visit	
Tests Done	
Diagnosis	
Treatment	
Mediction	
SHOT / VACCINATIONS	
WEIGHT	

Vet Visits

Date	
Vet Name	
E-Mail	
Phone	
Reason For Visit	
Tests Done	
Diagnosis	
Treatment	
Mediction	
SHOT / VACCINATIONS	
WEIGHT	

Vet Visits

Date	
Vet Name	
E-Mail	
Phone	
Reason For Visit	
Tests Done	
Diagnosis	
Treatment	
Mediction	
SHOT / VACCINATIONS	
WEIGHT	

Vet Visits

Date	
Vet Name	
E-Mail	
Phone	
Reason For Visit	
Tests Done	
Diagnosis	
Treatment	
Mediction	
SHOT / VACCINATIONS	
WEIGHT	

Vet Visits

Date	
Vet Name	
E-Mail	
Phone	
Reason For Visit	
Tests Done	
Diagnosis	
Treatment	
Mediction	
SHOT / VACCINATIONS	
WEIGHT	

Vet Visits

Date	
Vet Name	
E-Mail	
Phone	
Reason For Visit	
Tests Done	
Diagnosis	
Treatment	
Mediction	
SHOT / VACCINATIONS	
WEIGHT	

Vet Visits

Date	
Vet Name	
E-Mail	
Phone	
Reason For Visit	
Tests Done	
Diagnosis	
Treatment	
Mediction	
SHOT / VACCINATIONS	
WEIGHT	

Vet Visits

Date	
Vet Name	
E-Mail	
Phone	
Reason For Visit	
Tests Done	
Diagnosis	
Treatment	
Mediction	
SHOT / VACCINATIONS	
WEIGHT	

Vet Visits

Date	
Vet Name	
E-Mail	
Phone	
Reason For Visit	
Tests Done	
Diagnosis	
Treatment	
Mediction	
SHOT / VACCINATIONS	
WEIGHT	

Vet Visits	
Date	
Vet Name	
E-Mail	
Phone	
Reason For Visit	
Tests Done	
Diagnosis	
Treatment	
Med, Mediction	
SHOT / VACCINATIONS	
WEIGHT	

Vet Visits

Date	
Vet Name	
E-Mail	
Phone	
Reason For Visit	
Tests Done	
Diagnosis	
Treatment	
Mediction	
SHOT / VACCINATIONS	
WEIGHT	

Vet Visits

Date	
Vet Name	
E-Mail	
Phone	
Reason For Visit	
Tests Done	
Diagnosis	
Treatment	
Mediction	
SHOT / VACCINATIONS	
WEIGHT	

Vet Visits

Date	
Vet Name	
E-Mail	
Phone	
Reason For Visit	
Tests Done	
Diagnosis	
Treatment	
Mediction	
SHOT / VACCINATIONS	
WEIGHT	

Vet Visits

Date	
Vet Name	
E-Mail	
Phone	
Reason For Visit	
Tests Done	
Diagnosis	
Treatment	
Mediction	
SHOT / VACCINATIONS	
WEIGHT	

Vet Visits

Date	
Vet Name	
E-Mail	
Phone	
Reason For Visit	
Tests Done	
Diagnosis	
Treatment	
Mediction	
SHOT / VACCINATIONS	
WEIGHT	

Vet Visits

Date	
Vet Name	
E-Mail	
Phone	
Reason For Visit	
Tests Done	
Diagnosis	
Treatment	
Mediction	
SHOT / VACCINATIONS	
WEIGHT	

Vet Visits

Date	
Vet Name	
E-Mail	
Phone	
Reason For Visit	
Tests Done	
Diagnosis	
Treatment	
Mediction	
SHOT / VACCINATIONS	
WEIGHT	

Vet Visits

Date	
Vet Name	
E-Mail	
Phone	
Reason For Visit	
Tests Done	
Diagnosis	
Treatment	
Mediction	
SHOT / VACCINATIONS	
WEIGHT	

Vet Visits

Date	
Vet Name	
E-Mail	
Phone	
Reason For Visit	
Tests Done	
Diagnosis	
Treatment	
Mediction	
SHOT / VACCINATIONS	
WEIGHT	

Vet Visits

Date	
Vet Name	
E-Mail	
Phone	
Reason For Visit	
Tests Done	
Diagnosis	
Treatment	
Medriction	
SHOT / VACCINATIONS	
WEIGHT	

Vet Visits

Date	
Vet Name	
E-Mail	
Phone	
Reason For Visit	
Tests Done	
Diagnosis	
Treatment	
Mediction	
SHOT / VACCINATIONS	
WEIGHT	

Vet Visits

Date	
Vet Name	
E-Mail	
Phone	
Reason For Visit	
Tests Done	
Diagnosis	
Treatment	
Mediction	
SHOT / VACCINATIONS	
WEIGHT	

Vet Visits

Date	
Vet Name	
E-Mail	
Phone	
Reason For Visit	
Tests Done	
Diagnosis	
Treatment	
Mediction	
SHOT / VACCINATIONS	
WEIGHT	

Vet Visits

Date	
Vet Name	
E-Mail	
Phone	
Reason For Visit	
Tests Done	
Diagnosis	
Treatment	
Mediction	
SHOT / VACCINATIONS	
WEIGHT	

Vet Visits

Date	
Vet Name	
E-Mail	
Phone	
Reason For Visit	
Tests Done	
Diagnosis	
Treatment	
Mediction	
SHOT / VACCINATIONS	
WEIGHT	

Vet Visits

Date	
Vet Name	
E-Mail	
Phone	
Reason For Visit	
Tests Done	
Diagnosis	
Treatment	
Mediction	
SHOT / VACCINATIONS	
WEIGHT	

Vet Visits

Date	
Vet Name	
E-Mail	
Phone	
Reason For Visit	
Tests Done	
Diagnosis	
Treatment	
Mediction	
SHOT / VACCINATIONS	
WEIGHT	

Vet Visits

Date	
Vet Name	
E-Mail	
Phone	
Reason For Visit	
Tests Done	
Diagnosis	
Treatment	
Mediction	
SHOT / VACCINATIONS	
WEIGHT	

Vet Visits

Date	
Vet Name	
E-Mail	
Phone	
Reason For Visit	
Tests Done	
Diagnosis	
Treatment	
Mediction	
SHOT / VACCINATIONS	
WEIGHT	

Vet Visits

Date	
Vet Name	
E-Mail	
Phone	
Reason For Visit	
Tests Done	
Diagnosis	
Treatment	
Medction	
SHOT / VACCINATIONS	
WEIGHT	

Vet Visits

Date	
Vet Name	
E-Mail	
Phone	
Reason For Visit	
Tests Done	
Diagnosis	
Treatment	
Mediction	
SHOT / VACCINATIONS	
WEIGHT	

Vet Visits

Date	
Vet Name	
E-Mail	
Phone	
Reason For Visit	
Tests Done	
Diagnosis	
Treatment	
Mediction	
SHOT / VACCINATIONS	
WEIGHT	

Vet Visits

Date	
Vet Name	
E-Mail	
Phone	
Reason For Visit	
Tests Done	
Diagnosis	
Treatment	
Mediction	
SHOT / VACCINATIONS	
WEIGHT	

Vet Visits	
Date	
Vet Name	
E-Mail	
Phone	
Reason For Visit	
Tests Done	
Diagnosis	
Treatment	
Mediction	
SHOT / VACCINATIONS	
WEIGHT	

Vet Visits

Date	
Vet Name	
E-Mail	
Phone	
Reason For Visit	
Tests Done	
Diagnosis	
Treatment	
Mediction	
SHOT / VACCINATIONS	
WEIGHT	

Vet Visits	
Date	
Vet Name	
E-Mail	
Phone	
Reason For Visit	
Tests Done	
Diagnosis	
Treatment	
Mediction	
SHOT / VACCINATIONS	
WEIGHT	

Vet Visits

Date	
Vet Name	
E-Mail	
Phone	
Reason For Visit	
Tests Done	
Diagnosis	
Treatment	
Mediction	
SHOT / VACCINATIONS	
WEIGHT	

Vet Visits

Date	
Vet Name	
E-Mail	
Phone	
Reason For Visit	
Tests Done	
Diagnosis	
Treatment	
Mediction	
SHOT / VACCINATIONS	
WEIGHT	

Vet Visits

Date	
Vet Name	
E-Mail	
Phone	
Reason For Visit	
Tests Done	
Diagnosis	
Treatment	
Mediction	
SHOT / VACCINATIONS	
WEIGHT	

Vet Visits

Date	
Vet Name	
E-Mail	
Phone	
Reason For Visit	
Tests Done	
Diagnosis	
Treatment	
Mediction	
SHOT / VACCINATIONS	
WEIGHT	

Vet Visits

Date	
Vet Name	
E-Mail	
Phone	
Reason For Visit	
Tests Done	
Diagnosis	
Treatment	
Mediction	
SHOT / VACCINATIONS	
WEIGHT	

Vet Visits

Date	
Vet Name	
E-Mail	
Phone	
Reason For Visit	
Tests Done	
Diagnosis	
Treatment	
Mediction	
SHOT / VACCINATIONS	
WEIGHT	

Vet Visits

Date	
Vet Name	
E-Mail	
Phone	
Reason For Visit	
Tests Done	
Diagnosis	
Treatment	
Mediction	
SHOT / VACCINATIONS	
WEIGHT	

Vet Visits

Date	
Vet Name	
E-Mail	
Phone	
Reason For Visit	
Tests Done	
Diagnosis	
Treatment	
Mediction	
SHOT / VACCINATIONS	
WEIGHT	

Vet Visits

Date	
Vet Name	
E-Mail	
Phone	
Reason For Visit	
Tests Done	
Diagnosis	
Treatment	
Mediction	
SHOT / VACCINATIONS	
WEIGHT	

Vet Visits	
Date	
Vet Name	
E-Mail	
Phone	
Reason For Visit	
Tests Done	
Diagnosis	
Treatment	
Mediction	
SHOT / VACCINATIONS	
WEIGHT	

Vet Visits

Date	
Vet Name	
E-Mail	
Phone	
Reason For Visit	
Tests Done	
Diagnosis	
Treatment	
Mediction	
SHOT / VACCINATIONS	
WEIGHT	

Vet Visits

Date	
Vet Name	
E-Mail	
Phone	
Reason For Visit	
Tests Done	
Diagnosis	
Treatment	
Mediction	
SHOT / VACCINATIONS	
WEIGHT	

Vet Visits

Date	
Vet Name	
E-Mail	
Phone	
Reason For Visit	
Tests Done	
Diagnosis	
Treatment	
Mediction	
SHOT / VACCINATIONS	
WEIGHT	

Vet Visits

Date	
Vet Name	
E-Mail	
Phone	
Reason For Visit	
Tests Done	
Diagnosis	
Treatment	
Mediction	
SHOT / VACCINATIONS	
WEIGHT	

Vet Visits

Date	
Vet Name	
E-Mail	
Phone	
Reason For Visit	
Tests Done	
Diagnosis	
Treatment	
Mediction	
SHOT / VACCINATIONS	
WEIGHT	

Vet Visits	
Date	
Vet Name	
E-Mail	
Phone	
Reason For Visit	
Tests Done	
Diagnosis	
Treatment	
Mediction	
SHOT / VACCINATIONS	
WEIGHT	

Vet Visits

Date	
Vet Name	
E-Mail	
Phone	
Reason For Visit	
Tests Done	
Diagnosis	
Treatment	
Mediction	
SHOT / VACCINATIONS	
WEIGHT	

Vet Visits

Date	
Vet Name	
E-Mail	
Phone	
Reason For Visit	
Tests Done	
Diagnosis	
Treatment	
Mediction	
SHOT / VACCINATIONS	
WEIGHT	

Vet Visits

Date	
Vet Name	
E-Mail	
Phone	
Reason For Visit	
Tests Done	
Diagnosis	
Treatment	
Mediction	
SHOT / VACCINATIONS	
WEIGHT	

Vet Visits

Date	
Vet Name	
E-Mail	
Phone	
Reason For Visit	
Tests Done	
Diagnosis	
Treatment	
Mediction	
SHOT / VACCINATIONS	
WEIGHT	

Vet Visits

Date	
Vet Name	
E-Mail	
Phone	
Reason For Visit	
Tests Done	
Diagnosis	
Treatment	
Mediction	
SHOT / VACCINATIONS	
WEIGHT	

Vet Visits

Date	
Vet Name	
E-Mail	
Phone	
Reason For Visit	
Tests Done	
Diagnosis	
Treatment	
Mediction	
SHOT / VACCINATIONS	
WEIGHT	

Vet Visits

Date	
Vet Name	
E-Mail	
Phone	
Reason For Visit	
Tests Done	
Diagnosis	
Treatment	
Mediction	
SHOT / VACCINATIONS	
WEIGHT	

Vet Visits

Date	
Vet Name	
E-Mail	
Phone	
Reason For Visit	
Tests Done	
Diagnosis	
Treatment	
Mediction	
SHOT / VACCINATIONS	
WEIGHT	

Vet Visits

Date	
Vet Name	
E-Mail	
Phone	
Reason For Visit	
Tests Done	
Diagnosis	
Treatment	
Mediction	
SHOT / VACCINATIONS	
WEIGHT	

Vet Visits	
Date	
Vet Name	
E-Mail	
Phone	
Reason For Visit	
Tests Done	
Diagnosis	
Treatment	
Mediction	
SHOT / VACCINATIONS	
WEIGHT	

Vet Visits

Date	
Vet Name	
E-Mail	
Phone	
Reason For Visit	
Tests Done	
Diagnosis	
Treatment	
Mediction	
SHOT / VACCINATIONS	
WEIGHT	

Vet Visits

Date	
Vet Name	
E-Mail	
Phone	
Reason For Visit	
Tests Done	
Diagnosis	
Treatment	
Mediction	
SHOT / VACCINATIONS	
WEIGHT	

Vet Visits

Date	
Vet Name	
E-Mail	
Phone	
Reason For Visit	
Tests Done	
Diagnosis	
Treatment	
Mediction	
SHOT / VACCINATIONS	
WEIGHT	

Vet Visits

Date	
Vet Name	
E-Mail	
Phone	
Reason For Visit	
Tests Done	
Diagnosis	
Treatment	
Mediction	
SHOT / VACCINATIONS	
WEIGHT	

Vet Visits

Date	
Vet Name	
E-Mail	
Phone	
Reason For Visit	
Tests Done	
Diagnosis	
Treatment	
Mediction	
SHOT / VACCINATIONS	
WEIGHT	

Vet Visits	
Date	
Vet Name	
E-Mail	
Phone	
Reason For Visit	
Tests Done	
Diagnosis	
Treatment	
Mediction	
SHOT / VACCINATIONS	
WEIGHT	

Vet Visits

Date	
Vet Name	
E-Mail	
Phone	
Reason For Visit	
Tests Done	
Diagnosis	
Treatment	
Mediction	
SHOT / VACCINATIONS	
WEIGHT	

Vet Visits

Date	
Vet Name	
E-Mail	
Phone	
Reason For Visit	
Tests Done	
Diagnosis	
Treatment	
Mediction	
SHOT / VACCINATIONS	
WEIGHT	

Vet Visits

Date	
Vet Name	
E-Mail	
Phone	
Reason For Visit	
Tests Done	
Diagnosis	
Treatment	
Mediction	
SHOT / VACCINATIONS	
WEIGHT	

Vet Visits

Date	
Vet Name	
E-Mail	
Phone	
Reason For Visit	
Tests Done	
Diagnosis	
Treatment	
Mediction	
SHOT / VACCINATIONS	
WEIGHT	

Vet Visits

Date	
Vet Name	
E-Mail	
Phone	
Reason For Visit	
Tests Done	
Diagnosis	
Treatment	
Mediction	
SHOT / VACCINATIONS	
WEIGHT	

Vet Visits

Date	
Vet Name	
E-Mail	
Phone	
Reason For Visit	
Tests Done	
Diagnosis	
Treatment	
Mediction	
SHOT / VACCINATIONS	
WEIGHT	

Vet Visits

Date	
Vet Name	
E-Mail	
Phone	
Reason For Visit	
Tests Done	
Diagnosis	
Treatment	
Mediction	
SHOT / VACCINATIONS	
WEIGHT	

Vet Visits

Date	
Vet Name	
E-Mail	
Phone	
Reason For Visit	
Tests Done	
Diagnosis	
Treatment	
Mediction	
SHOT / VACCINATIONS	
WEIGHT	

Vet Visits

Date	
Vet Name	
E-Mail	
Phone	
Reason For Visit	
Tests Done	
Diagnosis	
Treatment	
Mediction	
SHOT / VACCINATIONS	
WEIGHT	

Vet Visits

Date	
Vet Name	
E-Mail	
Phone	
Reason For Visit	
Tests Done	
Diagnosis	
Treatment	
Mediction	
SHOT / VACCINATIONS	
WEIGHT	

Vet Visits

Date	
Vet Name	
E-Mail	
Phone	
Reason For Visit	
Tests Done	
Diagnosis	
Treatment	
Mediction	
SHOT / VACCINATIONS	
WEIGHT	

Vet Visits

Date	
Vet Name	
E-Mail	
Phone	
Reason For Visit	
Tests Done	
Diagnosis	
Treatment	
Mediction	
SHOT / VACCINATIONS	
WEIGHT	

Vet Visits

Date	
Vet Name	
E-Mail	
Phone	
Reason For Visit	
Tests Done	
Diagnosis	
Treatment	
Mediction	
SHOT / VACCINATIONS	
WEIGHT	

Vet Visits

Date	
Vet Name	
E-Mail	
Phone	
Reason For Visit	
Tests Done	
Diagnosis	
Treatment	
Mediction	
SHOT / VACCINATIONS	
WEIGHT	

Vet Visits

Date	
Vet Name	
E-Mail	
Phone	
Reason For Visit	
Tests Done	
Diagnosis	
Treatment	
Mediction	
SHOT / VACCINATIONS	
WEIGHT	

Vet Visits

Date	
Vet Name	
E-Mail	
Phone	
Reason For Visit	
Tests Done	
Diagnosis	
Treatment	
Medictíon	
SHOT / VACCINATIONS	
WEIGHT	

Vet Visits

Date	
Vet Name	
E-Mail	
Phone	
Reason For Visit	
Tests Done	
Diagnosis	
Treatment	
Mediction	
SHOT / VACCINATIONS	
WEIGHT	

Vet Visits

Date	
Vet Name	
E-Mail	
Phone	
Reason For Visit	
Tests Done	
Diagnosis	
Treatment	
Mediction	
SHOT / VACCINATIONS	
WEIGHT	

Vet Visits

Date	
Vet Name	
E-Mail	
Phone	
Reason For Visit	
Tests Done	
Diagnosis	
Treatment	
Mediction	
SHOT / VACCINATIONS	
WEIGHT	

Vet Visits

Date	
Vet Name	
E-Mail	
Phone	
Reason For Visit	
Tests Done	
Diagnosis	
Treatment	
Mediction	
SHOT / VACCINATIONS	
WEIGHT	

Vet Visits

Date	
Vet Name	
E-Mail	
Phone	
Reason For Visit	
Tests Done	
Diagnosis	
Treatment	
Mediction	
SHOT / VACCINATIONS	
WEIGHT	

Vet Visits	
Date	
Vet Name	
E-Mail	
Phone	
Reason For Visit	
Tests Done	
Diagnosis	
Treatment	
Mediction	
SHOT / VACCINATIONS	
WEIGHT	

Vet Visits

Date	
Vet Name	
E-Mail	
Phone	
Reason For Visit	
Tests Done	
Diagnosis	
Treatment	
Mediction	
SHOT / VACCINATIONS	
WEIGHT	

Vet Visits

Date	
Vet Name	
E-Mail	
Phone	
Reason For Visit	
Tests Done	
Diagnosis	
Treatment	
Medication	
SHOT / VACCINATIONS	
WEIGHT	

Vet Visits

Date	
Vet Name	
E-Mail	
Phone	
Reason For Visit	
Tests Done	
Diagnosis	
Treatment	
Mediction	
SHOT / VACCINATIONS	
WEIGHT	

Vet Visits

Date	
Vet Name	
E-Mail	
Phone	
Reason For Visit	
Tests Done	
Diagnosis	
Treatment	
Mediction	
SHOT / VACCINATIONS	
WEIGHT	

Vet Visits

Date	
Vet Name	
E-Mail	
Phone	
Reason For Visit	
Tests Done	
Diagnosis	
Treatment	
Mediction	
SHOT / VACCINATIONS	
WEIGHT	

Vet Visits

Date	
Vet Name	
E-Mail	
Phone	
Reason For Visit	
Tests Done	
Diagnosis	
Treatment	
Medication	
SHOT / VACCINATIONS	
WEIGHT	

Vet Visits

Date	
Vet Name	
E-Mail	
Phone	
Reason For Visit	
Tests Done	
Diagnosis	
Treatment	
Mediction	
SHOT / VACCINATIONS	
WEIGHT	

Vet Visits

Date	
Vet Name	
E-Mail	
Phone	
Reason For Visit	
Tests Done	
Diagnosis	
Treatment	
Mediction	
SHOT / VACCINATIONS	
WEIGHT	

Vet Visits

Date	
Vet Name	
E-Mail	
Phone	
Reason For Visit	
Tests Done	
Diagnosis	
Treatment	
Mediction	
SHOT / VACCINATIONS	
WEIGHT	

Note

Note

Note

Note

Note

Note

Note

Note

Note

Note

Made in the USA
Monee, IL
24 October 2021